# THE ULTIMATE
# HASHIMOTO AIP COOKBOOK

## Easy AIP Recipes for Hashimoto's Disease with 2-Week Action Meal Plan.

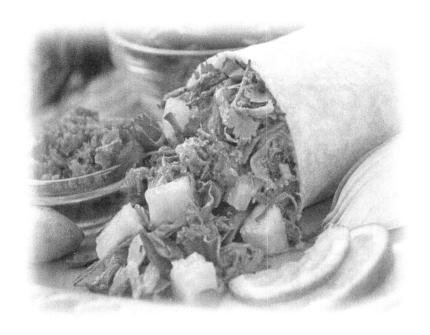

## CHRISTIANA WHITE

## GAIN ACCESS TO MORE BOOKS

# TABLE OF CONTENTS.

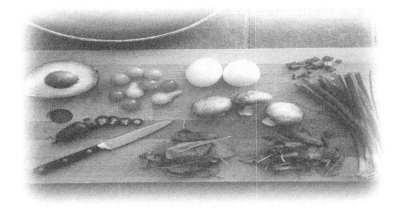

# INTRODUCTION

The heart of every kitchen contains a potential source of relief for people suffering with Hashimoto's disease. Welcome to the Hashimoto's Autoimmune Protocol Cookbook, where healthy recipes meet strong treatments. Countless people have found greater energy, fewer symptoms, and a more delicious approach to recovery in these pages.

This cookbook is more than simply a compilation of dishes; it's a guide and companion on your path to treating Hashimoto's symptoms. Join the community of people who have embraced the ideals outlined in these pages and discovered a road to vitality. From AIP basics to delectable recipes, this book is a road map to wellness in every mouthful.

Welcome to anyone looking for a tasty and inspiring method to manage their Hashimoto's. May this cookbook help you restore your health and enjoy the benefits of a healthy lifestyle.

# CHAPTER 1

## Understanding Hashimoto's and AIP Diet

Hashimoto's thyroiditis is an autoimmune disorder in which the immune system attacks the thyroid gland, resulting in low thyroid hormone levels and symptoms including fatigue, weight gain, hair loss, depression, and others. Hashimoto's disease is the most frequent cause of hypothyroidism in the United States, affecting approximately 5% of the population.

The AIP diet, also known as the autoimmune protocol diet, is a paleo-inspired diet that aims to reduce inflammation and repair the gut by removing foods that may cause or worsen inflammatory reactions. The AIP diet is based on the notion that leaky gut syndrome, or increased intestinal permeability, plays a significant role in the development and progression of autoimmune disorders.

The two stages of the AIP diet are reintroduction and elimination. Grains, legumes, dairy, eggs, nuts, seeds, nightshades, gluten, sugar, alcohol, caffeine, and processed oils are among items that should be avoided during the elimination period.

During the reintroduction phase, some of the excluded foods are progressively added back one at a time while monitoring for any adverse responses.

The AIP diet may help persons with Hashimoto's disease by lowering thyroid antibodies, inflammation, and symptoms while also increasing thyroid function, hormone levels, and overall quality of life. However, the AIP diet is not a cure for Hashimoto's and should be taken as a supplement to medicine and other lifestyle changes.

## The Link between Hashimoto's Disease and the Autoimmune Protocol

The autoimmune protocol diet and Hashimoto's disease are linked because the gut-immune axis, or the connection of the gut bacteria, the intestinal barrier, and the immune system, is thought to impact both disorders. The gut-immune axis is critical for maintaining immunological homeostasis and avoiding autoimmune reactions.

However, genetic predisposition, environmental triggers, infections, stress, and food can all disturb the gut-immune axis, resulting in increased intestinal permeability, dysbiosis, and inflammation. This can activate self-reactive immune cells and cause the creation of autoantibodies against the thyroid gland or other organs.

The autoimmune protocol diet seeks to heal the gut-immune axis by eliminating potential dietary triggers and encouraging the growth of beneficial bacteria. The AIP diet may potentially influence the immune system by decreasing pro-inflammatory cytokines and increasing anti-inflammatory cytokines, as well as improving regulatory T cells that suppress autoimmune reactions.

Some studies have found that the AIP diet can improve clinical outcomes and quality of life in persons suffering from Hashimoto's and other autoimmune disorders such inflammatory bowel disease, rheumatoid arthritis, multiple sclerosis, and psoriasis.

However, further research is needed to establish the AIP diet's efficacy and safety for autoimmune illnesses, as well as to understand the processes underlying its effectiveness.

# CHAPTER 2

## Foods to Include on the AIP Diet

The AIP diet allows and encourages the following foods:

- Lean meat, chicken, and fish.
- Organ meats and bone broth.
- Vegetables (except nightshades).
- Fruits (with moderation)
- Healthy fats (such as coconut oil, olive oil, and avocado oil).
- Fermented foods (such as sauerkraut, kimchi, and kombucha).
- Herbs and spices (except those made from seeds or nightshades)
- Vinegar with lemon juice
- Honey, maple syrup (in moderation)

## Foods to avoid in the AIP Diet

The AIP diet avoids the following foods:

- Grains, legumes, and pseudograins.
- Dairy and Eggs
- Nuts & seeds

- Nightshades, which include eggplants, tomatoes, potatoes, and peppers.
- Gluten-free grains
- Refined sugar and artificial sweeteners.
- Processed oils and fats.
- Alcohol and Caffeine
- Spices made from seeds or nightshades.
- Food additives and preservatives.

## The Elimination and Reintroduction Phase

The AIP diet consists of two phases: elimination and reintroduction. The elimination phase entails avoiding all of the foods mentioned above for at least 30 days, or until symptoms improve.

During the reintroduction phase, some of the excluded foods are progressively added back one at a time while monitoring for any adverse responses.

This stage can assist detect particular food intolerances and tailor the diet to one's specific needs and preferences.

# CHAPTER 3

## Cooking Methods for Preserving Nutritional Value

The nutritional content of food can be influenced by a variety of factors, including the kind, quality, and freshness of the ingredients, as well as the cooking method, temperature, duration, and water quantity utilized.

Some cooking methods improve the flavor, texture, and digestibility of food, whereas others diminish or eliminate vitamins, minerals, antioxidants, and phytochemicals that are good to health.

Here are some general suggestions for preserving the nutritional content of food while cooking:

- Use fresh, organic, and seasonal ingredients whenever possible.
- Wash, peel, and cut fruits and vegetables right before cooking to reduce nutrient loss.
- Use a sharp knife and avoid over-chopping or shredding fruits and vegetables because this exposes more surface area to oxygen and heat.
- Cook fruits and vegetables with their skins on, which contain fiber and antioxidants.

- To prevent leaching and degradation of water-soluble nutrients, such as vitamin C and B vitamins, use as little water as possible and cook for the least amount of time.
- Use the cooking water in soups, sauces, or gravies to preserve the nutrients that have dissolved into it.
- Avoid adding baking soda to veggies since it can damage vitamin C and decrease the availability of minerals.
- Avoid deep-frying, which can increase the fat and calorie content of food while also producing hazardous substances like acrylamide and Trans fats.
- Use healthy oils, such as olive, avocado, or coconut oil, and avoid overheating them, as they may lose their nutritional content and release free radicals.
- To improve the taste of food, use herbs, spices, vinegar, lemon juice, or other natural flavourings instead of salt, sugar, or artificial additives.
- To avoid spoiling and bacterial growth, store cooked foods in airtight containers and refrigerate or freeze them as soon as feasible.

**Some of the greatest cooking techniques to preserve the nutritional value of food are:**

• Steaming: Instead of immersing food in water, this method cooks it using hot steam. It is perfect for delicate foods like fish, seafood, and vegetables since it retains their original flavor, color, and texture.

Steaming also preserves the majority of water-soluble and heat-sensitive nutrients, including vitamin C, folate, and thiamine, as well as antioxidants and phytochemicals that protect against oxidative stress and inflammation.

• Sautéing and stir-frying: These techniques employ a tiny amount of oil and high heat to cook food rapidly and evenly in a skillet or wok. They are ideal for meats, poultry, eggs, and vegetables because they seal in the fluids and flavor of the food while browning the surface and generating a crispy texture. Sautéing and stir-frying also keep most nutrients, especially when the food is sliced into small pieces and cooked quickly.

However, avoid burning or overcooking the food, since this can diminish the vitamin C and B vitamin content while also producing hazardous substances like acrylamide and heterocyclic amines.

• Roasting and Baking: These techniques employ dry heat in an oven to cook food slowly and completely. They are excellent for meats, poultry, fish, and root vegetables, enhancing their flavor, tenderness, and juiciness while forming a golden crust.

Roasting and baking also retain the majority of fat-soluble nutrients, including vitamin A, vitamin D, vitamin E, and vitamin K, as well as minerals like iron, zinc, and selenium.

However, roasting and baking at high temperatures can lower vitamin C and B vitamin concentrations while also producing hazardous substances like acrylamide and heterocyclic amines.

• Microwaving: This method employs electromagnetic waves to heat and cook food quickly and evenly. It is both convenient and energy-efficient, and may be used to prepare a wide range of items, including meats, poultry, eggs, vegetables, and cereals. Microwaving protects the majority of nutrients, particularly the water-soluble and heat-sensitive ones, because it requires little water and time.

Microwaving, on the other hand, can affect the texture, color, and flavor of some foods, as well as release hazardous substances like acrylamide and heterocyclic amines if the food is overheated or heated in plastic containers.

# Essential Kitchen Tools for AIP Cooking.

To effectively follow the AIP diet, you'll need several key kitchen gear that make cooking easier and more fun. Some of the important kitchen tools for AIP cuisine are:

• An excellent chef's knife: A sharp and durable knife is essential for chopping, slicing, and dicing fruits, vegetables, meats, and herbs. A excellent chef's knife may help you prepare meals faster and safer, while also reducing waste and nutrient loss.

A good chef's knife should be ergonomic, well-balanced, and simple to sharpen.

• A cutting board is a flat surface that protects both the countertop and the knife blade from injury. A cutting board should be large enough to hold the food being sliced and made of a durable, non-porous material like wood, bamboo, or plastic.

Clean and sterilize a cutting board after each use, and replace it if it becomes worn or broken.

• A Slow Cooker: A slow cooker is an electric device that cooks food at a low and consistent temperature for several hours. A slow cooker is perfect for creating soups, stews, casseroles, and roasts because it retains the flavor, moisture, and nutrients of the meal while tenderizing tough cuts of meat.

A slow cooker is also convenient and energy-efficient, as it cooks meals without monitoring and consumes less electricity than an oven.

• A Pressure Cooker: A sealed pot that cooks food using high pressure and steam. A pressure cooker is perfect for creating bone broth, soups, stews, and roasts since it decreases cooking time while increasing the flavor and nutrient content of the food.

A pressure cooker is also practical and energy-efficient because it cooks food faster and consumes less water and electricity than a traditional pot.

• A Spiralizer: A spiralizer is a tool for transforming vegetables into long, thin noodles or ribbons. A spiralizer is perfect for producing veggie pasta, salads, and stir-fries since it adds variety, texture, and color to the foods while also improving fiber and antioxidant consumption.

A spiralizer can also assist limit your intake of grains and gluten, which are prohibited on the AIP diet.

• A Food Processor: A food processor is an electrical device that chops, slices, shreds, grinds, purees, and mixes food. A food processor is perfect for preparing sauces, dips, pesto, hummus, nut butters, and baked products since it saves time and produces smooth and consistent results.

A food processor can also assist enhance your intake of fruits, veggies, and healthy fats, all of which are recommended on the AIP diet.

• A Blender: A blender is an electric appliance used to liquefy and mix food. A blender is perfect for producing smoothies, soups, sauces, and dressings since it produces creamy and foamy textures while blending various flavors and ingredients.

A blender can also help you consume more fruits, veggies, and liquids, all of which are good for your health and digestion.

# CHAPTER 4

## Breakfast Recipes

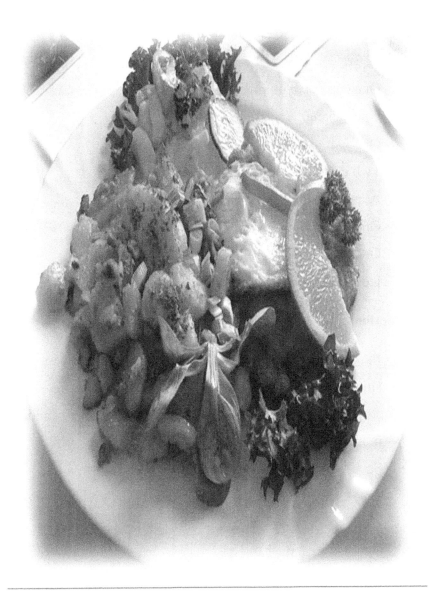

# AIP Green Smoothie

**Servings: two.**

**Prepare time: 5 minutes.**

**Ingredients:**

- One cup coconut milk.
- One banana.
- One-half avocado
- Two cups baby spinach.
- A quarter cup of fresh mint leaves
- One spoonful of honey.
- One teaspoon of vanilla extract.
- Ice cubes, as needed.

**Instructions:**

- In a blender, combine all the ingredients and process until smooth and creamy.
- Adjust the sweetness and thickness to your liking by adding more honey or ice.
- Savor your delicious and nutritious smoothie!

# Coconut Flour Pancakes.

**Servings: four.**

**Prep time is 10 minutes.**

**Cook for 15 minutes.**

**Ingredients:**

- One-quarter cup coconut flour
- One-quarter teaspoon of baking soda
- One pinch of salt.
- 4 eggs
- 1/4 cup melted coconut oil.
- One-quarter cup coconut milk
- One spoonful of honey.
- One teaspoon of vanilla extract.
- Coconut oil for frying.

**Instructions:**

- In a large bowl, combine the coconut flour, baking soda, and salt.
- In a separate dish, whisk together the eggs, coconut oil, coconut milk, honey, and vanilla extract.
- Combine the wet and dry ingredients and mix thoroughly to create a smooth batter.

- Place a skillet over medium-high heat and coat it with coconut oil.
- Pour about 1/4 cup batter into the skillet and heat for 3 minutes, or until bubbles appear on the surface.
- Flip the pancake and cook for a further 2 minutes, or until golden and cooked through.
- Repeat with the remaining batter, using extra coconut oil as needed.
- Top your pancakes with your favorite ingredients, including fresh berries, coconut whipped cream, or maple syrup.

## Sweet Potato Hash

**Servings: four.**

**Prepare time: 15 minutes.**

**Cook for 25 minutes.**

**Ingredients:**

- Four medium sweet potatoes, peeled and diced
- Two teaspoons of coconut oil.
- Add salt and pepper to taste.
- 4 bacon pieces, chopped
- 1 onion, chopped

- 2 garlic cloves, minced
- Two cups baby spinach.
- Fresh parsley to garnish.

**Instructions:**

- Preheat the oven to 400°F. Use parchment paper to line a baking sheet.
- Toss the sweet potatoes with 1 tablespoon coconut oil, salt, and pepper, then distribute them evenly on the prepared baking sheet.
- Bake for 20 minutes, or until soft and golden. Flip halfway through.
- Cook the bacon in a large skillet over medium-high heat, stirring periodically, until crisp, about 15 minutes. Transfer to a dish lined with paper towels and set aside.
- In the same skillet, heat the remaining coconut oil and cook the onion and garlic until tender, about 10 minutes. Season with salt and pepper to taste.
- Cook for about 5 minutes, or until the spinach has wilted.
- Place the sweet potatoes on a big plate and top with the onion-spinach mixture and bacon. Sprinkle with parsley and serve.

# AIP Breakfast Casserole

**Servings: six.**

**Prep time is 10 minutes.**

**Cook for 40 minutes.**

**Ingredients:**

- One pound of ground pork.
- One teaspoon of dried sage.
- 1/2 teaspoon dried thyme.
- One-quarter teaspoon of salt
- 1/4 teaspoon black pepper.
- Two teaspoons of coconut oil.
- 1 onion, diced
- 2 Cups of broccoli florets, chopped
- Two cups cauliflower rice.
- One-quarter cup coconut milk
- One-quarter cup nutritional yeast
- One-quarter teaspoon of garlic powder
- One-quarter teaspoon of onion powder
- Fresh parsley to garnish.

**Instructions:**

- Preheat the oven to 375°F. Grease a 9x13-inch baking dish.
- In a large mixing bowl, combine the pork, sage, thyme, salt, and pepper. Form tiny patties and set aside.
- Heat the coconut oil in a big skillet over medium-high heat. Cook the patties for about 15 minutes, or until browned on both sides. Transfer to the prepared baking dish and set aside.
- In the same skillet, cook the onion until tender, about 10 minutes. Cook the broccoli and cauliflower rice until soft, about 10 minutes. Season with salt and pepper to taste.
- In a small mixing dish, combine the coconut milk, nutritional yeast, garlic powder, and onion powder. Pour over the broccoli-cauliflower mixture. Stir to blend, then pour equally over the pork patties in the baking dish.
- Bake for 15 minutes, until bubbling and golden.
- Sprinkle with parsley and serve.

# Banana Cinnamon Muffins

**Serves: 12**

**Prep time is 10 minutes.**

**Cook for 25 minutes.**

**Ingredients:**

- 3 ripe bananas (mashed)
- 1/4 cup melted coconut oil.
- One-quarter cup honey
- One teaspoon of vanilla extract.
- One-quarter cup coconut flour
- 1/4 cup arrowroot starch.
- One-quarter teaspoon of baking soda
- One-quarter teaspoon of salt
- One teaspoon of cinnamon.
- Coconut oil for greasing.

**Instructions:**

- Preheat the oven to 350°F. Use coconut oil to grease a 12-cup muffin tray.
- In a large mixing bowl, blend the bananas, coconut oil, honey, and vanilla essence until thoroughly incorporated.

- In a small bowl, combine the coconut flour, arrowroot starch, baking soda, salt, and cinnamon.
- Combine the dry ingredients with the wet components and mix thoroughly to produce a homogeneous batter.
- Divide the batter evenly among the prepared muffin cups, filling each about 3/4 full.
- When a toothpick inserted in the center comes out clean, bake for 20 to 25 minutes.
- Allow the muffins to cool briefly in the pan before transferring to a wire rack to cool entirely.
- Enjoy your lovely, fluffy muffins!

## AIP Porridge

**Servings: two.**

**Prepare time: 5 minutes.**

**Cook for 10 minutes.**

**Ingredients:**

- One-quarter cup coconut flour
- Two teaspoons of gelatin.
- Two glasses of water.
- One-quarter cup coconut milk

- Two teaspoons of honey.
- One-fourth teaspoon cinnamon
- Fresh berries for topping.

**Instructions:**

- In a small bowl, whisk together the coconut flour and gelatin until thoroughly incorporated.
- Heat the water in a small saucepan over medium heat until it boils.
- Slowly whisk in the coconut flour-gelatin mixture, whisking constantly to prevent lumps.
- Simmer for ten minutes over low heat, stirring frequently.
- Stir in the coconut milk, honey, and cinnamon, then adjust the sweetness and thickness to your liking.
- Serve your warm, creamy porridge with fresh berries on top.

# Sausage and Vegetable Skillet

**Servings: four.**

**Prep time is 10 minutes.**

**Cook for 20 minutes.**

**Ingredients:**

- One pound of ground pork.
- One teaspoon of dried sage.
- 1/2 teaspoon dried thyme.
- One-quarter teaspoon of salt
- 1/4 teaspoon black pepper.
- Two teaspoons of coconut oil.
- 1 onion, sliced
- 2 garlic cloves, minced
- 2 cups Brussels sprouts, halved
- 2 cups butternut squash, peeled and diced.
- Fresh parsley to garnish.

**Instructions**:

- In a large mixing bowl, combine the pork, sage, thyme, salt, and pepper. Form little balls and set aside.

- In a large skillet over medium-high heat, heat the coconut oil and brown the meatballs on both sides, about 15 minutes. Transfer to a dish to keep heated.
- In the same skillet, cook the onion and garlic until soft, about 10 minutes. Cook the Brussels sprouts and butternut squash until soft, about 10 minutes. Season with salt and pepper to taste.
- Return the meatballs to the skillet and stir them with the vegetables.
- Sprinkle with parsley and serve.

## AIP Breakfast Tacos

**Servings: four.**

**Prepare time: 15 minutes.**

**Cook for 15 minutes.**

**Ingredients:**

**Regarding the tortillas:**

- One-quarter cup coconut flour
- 1/4 cup arrowroot starch.
- One-quarter teaspoon of salt
- One-quarter cup water

- Two teaspoons of coconut oil.

**For the Filling:**

- One tablespoon of coconut oil.
- 1/2 lb ground beef.
- One-quarter teaspoon of salt
- 1/4 teaspoon black pepper.
- One-quarter teaspoon of garlic powder
- One-quarter teaspoon of onion powder
- 1/4 teaspoon oregano.
- One-quarter teaspoon of cumin
- One-quarter teaspoon of turmeric
- Two cups of shredded lettuce.
- 1/4 cup chopped cilantro.
- A quarter cup of coconut yogurt

**Instructions:**

- To create the tortillas, combine the coconut flour, arrowroot starch, and salt in a medium mixing basin. Add the water and coconut oil, and stir to produce a smooth dough.
- Divide the dough into eight equal sections, then roll each into a ball. Place each ball between two sheets of parchment paper and use a rolling pin or your hands to flatten into a thin circle.

- In a non-stick skillet over medium heat, cook each tortilla for about 2 minutes on each side, or until lightly browned and cooked through. Transfer to a dish to keep heated.
- To make the filling, in a big skillet, warm the coconut oil over medium-high heat. For around fifteen minutes, sauté the ground beef, breaking it up with a spatula, until it is browned and cooked through.
- Drain out any extra fat and season with salt, pepper, garlic powder, onion powder, oregano, cumin, and turmeric. Stir thoroughly to mix.
- To make the tacos, put part of the beef mixture onto each tortilla, then top with lettuce, cilantro, and coconut yogurt. Fold in half and enjoy!

# AIP Waffles

**Servings: four.**

**Prep time is 10 minutes.**

**Cook for 15 minutes.**

**• Ingredients:**

- One-quarter cup coconut flour
- 1/4 cup arrowroot starch.
- One-quarter teaspoon of baking soda
- One pinch of salt.
- 4 eggs
- 1/4 cup melted coconut oil.
- One-quarter cup coconut milk
- One spoonful of honey.
- One teaspoon of vanilla extract.
- Coconut oil for greasing.

**Instructions:**

- Preheat the waffle machine and grease it with coconut oil.
- In a large basin, combine the coconut flour, arrowroot starch, baking soda, and salt.
- In a separate dish, whisk together the eggs, coconut oil, coconut milk, honey, and vanilla extract.

- Combine the wet and dry ingredients and mix thoroughly to create a smooth batter.
- Pour approximately 1/4 cup batter into the waffle machine and cook for 3 to 4 minutes, or until golden and crisp.
- Repeat with the remaining batter, using extra coconut oil as needed.
- Top your waffles with your favorite ingredients, such as fresh berries, coconut whipped cream, or maple syrup.

## AIP Breakfast Burrito

**Servings: four.**

**Prepare time: 15 minutes.**

**Cook for 15 minutes.**

**Ingredients:**

**Regarding the tortillas:**

- One-quarter cup coconut flour
- 1/4 cup arrowroot starch.
- One-quarter teaspoon of salt
- One-quarter cup water
- Two teaspoons of coconut oil.

## For the Filling:

- One tablespoon of coconut oil.
- 1/2 pound ground turkey.
- One-quarter teaspoon of salt
- 1/4 teaspoon black pepper.
- One-quarter teaspoon of garlic powder
- One-quarter teaspoon of onion powder
- 1/4 teaspoon oregano.
- One-quarter teaspoon of turmeric
- Two cups of shredded cabbage.
- 1/4 cup chopped cilantro.
- A quarter cup of coconut yogurt

## Instructions:

- To create the tortillas, combine the coconut flour, arrowroot starch, and salt in a medium mixing basin. Add the water and coconut oil, and stir to produce a smooth dough.
- Divide the dough into eight equal sections, then roll each into a ball. Place each ball between two sheets of parchment paper and use a rolling pin or your hands to flatten into a thin circle.
- In a nonstick skillet over medium heat, cook each tortilla for about 2 minutes on each side, or until lightly browned and cooked through. Transfer to a dish to keep heated.

- To create the filling, in a big skillet, warm the coconut oil over medium-high heat. Cook the turkey, breaking it up with a spatula, until browned and cooked through, about 15 minutes.

- Drain out any extra fat and season with salt, pepper, garlic powder, onion powder, oregano, and turmeric. Stir thoroughly to mix.

- Cook the cabbage and cilantro for about 5 minutes, or until wilted.

- To assemble the burritos, pour some turkey-cabbage mixture onto each tortilla and top with coconut yogurt. Fold in the sides and roll tightly. Enjoy!

# CHAPTER 5

## Soup and Salad Recipes.

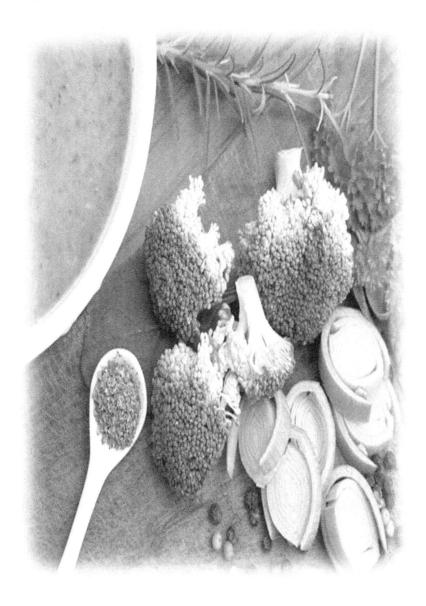

# AIP Chicken Soup

**Servings: six.**

**Prep time is 10 minutes.**

**Cook for 30 minutes.**

**Ingredients:**

- Two teaspoons of coconut oil.
- 1 onion, chopped
- Two carrots, peeled and sliced
- Two celery stalks, chopped
- 4 garlic cloves, minced
- One teaspoon dried thyme.
- One teaspoon of dried rosemary.
- One teaspoon of salt.
- Eight cups of chicken bone broth.
- 4 cups shredded cooked chicken.
- 2 tablespoons chopped parsley.

**Instructions:**

- In a large saucepan over medium-high heat, heat the coconut oil and sauté the onion, carrots, celery, garlic, thyme, rosemary, and salt until tender, about 15 minutes.

- Bring the chicken bone broth to a boil. Reduce the heat and let the vegetables to simmer for about 15 minutes, or until tender.
- Stir in the shredded chicken and parsley, and cook for about 5 minutes.
- Enjoy your warm, cozy soup!

## AIP Broccoli Soup

**Servings: four.**

**Prep time is 10 minutes.**

**Cook for 20 minutes.**

**Ingredients:**

- Two teaspoons of coconut oil.
- 1 onion, chopped
- Four cups of broccoli florets.
- Four cups of chicken bone broth.
- One-quarter cup coconut cream
- Add salt and pepper to taste.

**Instructions:**

- Heat the coconut oil in a large pot over medium-high heat, then sauté the onion until tender, about 10 minutes.
- Heat the broccoli and chicken bone broth together until boiling. Reduce the heat and let the broccoli to simmer for about 10 minutes, or until tender.
- Puree the soup in an immersion blender or normal blender until smooth and creamy.
- Stir in the coconut cream and season with salt and pepper as desired.
- Enjoy your creamy, nourishing soup!

## AIP Pumpkin Soup

**Servings: four.**

**Prep time is 10 minutes.**

**Cook for 25 minutes.**

**Ingredients:**

- Two teaspoons of coconut oil.
- 1 onion, chopped
- 2 garlic cloves, minced
- 4 cups pumpkin puree.

- Four cups of chicken bone broth.
- One-quarter cup coconut milk
- One teaspoon of cinnamon.
- 1/4 teaspoon nutmeg.
- Add salt and pepper to taste.

**Instructions**:

- Heat the coconut oil in a large pot over medium-high heat, then sauté the onion and garlic until tender, about 10 minutes.
- Heat the pumpkin puree and chicken bone broth together until boiling. Reduce the heat to a simmer for about 15 minutes, or until the pumpkin is well heated.
- Add the coconut milk, cinnamon, nutmeg, salt, and pepper to taste.
- Enjoy your warm, spicy soup!

## AIP Salad with Grilled Chicken

**Servings: four.**

**Prepare time: 15 minutes.**

**Cook for 15 minutes.**

**Ingredients:**

**For the Chicken:**

- Four chicken breasts.
- Two teaspoons of olive oil.
- Two teaspoons of apple cider vinegar.
- One teaspoon of dried oregano.
- One teaspoon dried basil.
- A half teaspoon of salt.
- 1/4 teaspoon black pepper (omit during the elimination phase of AIP)

**For the Salad:**

- Eight cups of mixed greens.
- 2 cups cherry tomatoes, halved
- One-quarter cup sliced black olives
- 1/4 cup chopped parsley.

**For dressing**:

- One-quarter cup olive oil
- Two teaspoons of apple cider vinegar.
- One teaspoon of honey.
- A half teaspoon of salt.
- 1/4 teaspoon black pepper (omit during the elimination phase of AIP)

**Instructions:**

- To prepare the chicken, place the breasts in a large ziplock bag with the olive oil, apple cider vinegar, oregano, basil, salt, and pepper.
- Chicken should be massaged to coat it in marinade once the bag is sealed. Put it in the fridge for at least half an hour or maybe overnight.
- Preheat a grill or grill pan over medium-high heat and cook the chicken for about 7 minutes on each side, or until cooked through and no longer pink in the middle.
- Transfer to a chopping board and let sit for 5 minutes. Slice thinly and set aside.
- To prepare the salad, combine the mixed greens, cherry tomatoes, black olives, and parsley in a big bowl.
- To create the dressing, combine the olive oil, apple cider vinegar, honey, salt, and pepper in a small bowl or jar.
- To serve, place the salad on four dishes and top with the sliced chicken. Drizzle with dressing and enjoy!

# AIP Greek Salad

**Servings: four.**

**Prepare time: 15 minutes.**

**Ingredients:**

**For the Salad:**

- Eight cups of chopped romaine lettuce.
- 2 cups cherry tomatoes, halved
- One-quarter cup sliced black olives
- 1/4 cup chopped parsley.

**For Dressing:**

- One-quarter cup olive oil
- Two teaspoons of apple cider vinegar.
- One teaspoon of dried oregano.
- A half teaspoon of salt.
- 1/4 teaspoon black pepper (omit during the elimination phase of AIP)

**Instructions:**

- To make the salad, combine the lettuce, tomatoes, olives, and parsley in a large bowl.
- To create the dressing, combine the olive oil, apple cider vinegar, oregano, salt, and pepper in a small bowl or jar.

- To serve, drizzle the salad with the dressing and dig in!

# AIP Coleslaw

**Servings: six.**

**Prepare time: 15 minutes.**

**Ingredients:**

**For coleslaw:**

- 4 cups shredded green cabbage.
- Two cups of shredded red cabbage.
- Two carrots, peeled and grated
- 2 green onions, sliced

**For Dressing:**

- 1/2 cup coconut yogurt.
- Two teaspoons of apple cider vinegar.
- One spoonful of honey.
- A half teaspoon of salt.
- 1/4 teaspoon black pepper (omit during the elimination phase of AIP)

**Instructions:**

- To make the coleslaw, combine the cabbage, carrots, and green onions in a large bowl.
- To make the dressing, combine the coconut yogurt, apple cider vinegar, honey, salt, and pepper in a small bowl or jar.
- To serve, combine the coleslaw and dressing, and enjoy!

## AIP Kale Salad

**Servings: four.**

**Prepare time: 15 minutes.**

**Ingredients:**

**For the Salad:**

- 8 cups of kale, trimmed and chopped
- Two teaspoons of lemon juice.
- Two teaspoons of olive oil.
- Add salt and pepper to taste.
- 1/4 cup raisins.
- One-quarter cup sunflower seeds

**For Dressing:**

- One-quarter cup coconut milk
- 2 tablespoons tahini (omit during the elimination phase of AIP)
- One spoonful of honey.
- One-quarter teaspoon of garlic powder
- Add salt and pepper to taste.

**Instructions:**

- In a large bowl, massage the kale with lemon juice, olive oil, salt, and pepper until it is wilted and tender, about 10 minutes.
- Toss in the raisins and sunflower seeds until combined.
- To prepare the dressing, combine the coconut milk, tahini, honey, garlic powder, salt, and pepper in a small bowl or jar.
- To serve, drizzle the salad with the dressing and dig in!

# AIP Beetroot Soup

**Servings: four.**

**Prep time is 10 minutes.**

**Cook for 25 minutes.**

**Ingredients:**

- Two teaspoons of coconut oil.
- 1 onion, chopped
- 4 cups peeled and diced beetroot.
- Four cups of veggie broth.
- Add salt and pepper to taste.
- One-quarter cup coconut cream
- Fresh dill as garnish

**Instructions:**

- Heat the coconut oil in a large pot over medium-high heat, then sauté the onion until tender, about 10 minutes.
- Bring the beets and vegetable broth to a boil. Reduce the heat and let the beetroot to simmer for about 15 minutes, or until tender.
- Puree the soup in an immersion blender or normal blender until smooth and velvety.
- Add salt and pepper to taste.

- Mix in the coconut cream and garnish with dill.
- Enjoy your vivid and flavorful soup!

# AIP Cucumber Salad

**Servings: four.**

**Prep time is 10 minutes.**

**Ingredients:**

- 4 cups sliced cucumbers.
- 1/4 cup chopped fresh mint.
- Two teaspoons of olive oil.
- Two teaspoons of apple cider vinegar.
- One teaspoon of honey.
- Add salt and pepper to taste.

**Instructions:**

- In a large bowl, combine the cucumbers and mint.
- In a small bowl or jar, combine olive oil, apple cider vinegar, honey, salt, and pepper.
- Pour the dressing over the cucumber salad and toss to coat.
- Savor your delicious and crispy salad!

# AIP Carrot Soup

**Servings: four.**

**Prep time is 10 minutes.**

**Cook for 20 minutes.**

**Ingredients:**

- Two teaspoons of coconut oil.
- 1 onion, chopped
- Four cups of carrots, peeled and sliced
- Four cups of chicken bone broth.
- One-quarter teaspoon ginger
- One-quarter teaspoon of turmeric
- Add salt and pepper to taste.
- One-quarter cup coconut cream
- Fresh cilantro to garnish.

**Instructions**:

- Heat the coconut oil in a large pot over medium-high heat, then sauté the onion until tender, about 10 minutes.
- Boil the carrots, chicken bone broth, ginger, turmeric, salt, and pepper. Reduce the heat and let the carrots simmer for about 10 minutes, or until soft.
- Puree the soup in an immersion blender or normal blender until smooth and creamy.
- Mix in the coconut cream and sprinkle with cilantro.
- Enjoy your warm, calming soup!

# CHAPTER 6

## Main Dish Recipes.

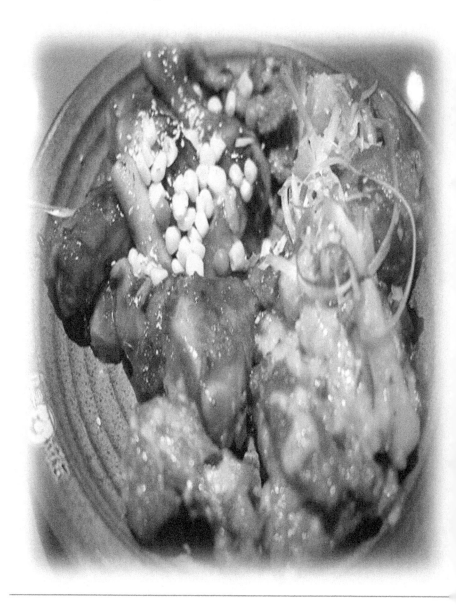

# AIP Chicken Stir-fry

**Servings: four.**

**Prepare time: 15 minutes.**

**Cook for 15 minutes.**

**Ingredients:**

- 1/4 cup coconut aminos.
- Two teaspoons of apple cider vinegar.
- One spoonful of honey.
- One teaspoon garlic powder.
- One teaspoon of ginger powder.
- One-quarter teaspoon of salt
- 1/4 teaspoon black pepper (omit during the elimination phase of AIP)
- 1/4 cup arrowroot starch.
- Cut 1 pound of chicken breast into bite-size pieces.
- Two teaspoons of coconut oil.
- Four cups of mixed veggies, including broccoli, carrots, zucchini, and mushrooms.
- 2 tablespoons sesame seeds (omit during the elimination phase of AIP)
- Fresh cilantro to garnish.

**Instructions:**

- In a small mixing bowl, combine the coconut aminos, apple cider vinegar, honey, garlic powder, ginger powder, salt, and pepper. Set aside.
- In a separate small bowl, mix the chicken with the arrowroot starch until thoroughly coated. Shake out any excess starch.
- Heat the coconut oil in a big skillet over high heat, then add the chicken and cook for about 10 minutes, tossing occasionally. Transfer to a dish to keep heated.
- In the same skillet, stir fried the mixed vegetables until crisp-tender, about 5 minutes.
- Return the chicken to the skillet and pour in the sauce. Stir to coat, then cook for about 2 minutes, or until the sauce thickens.
- Garnish with sesame seeds and cilantro and serve.

## AIP Beef Stew

**Servings: six.**

**Prepare time: 15 minutes.**

**Cook for 8 hours.**

**Ingredients:**

- Cut 2 pounds of beef chuck into 1-inch cubes.

- 1/4 cup arrowroot starch.
- One-quarter teaspoon of salt
- 1/4 teaspoon black pepper (omit during the elimination phase of AIP)
- Two teaspoons of coconut oil.
- Four cups of beef bone broth.
- Two teaspoons of apple cider vinegar.
- One tablespoon dried rosemary.
- One tablespoon dried thyme.
- Two bay leaves.
- 4 garlic cloves, minced
- 4 peeled and chopped carrots.
- Four celery stalks, chopped
- Two parsnips, peeled and chopped
- Fresh parsley to garnish.

**Instructions:**

- Toss the beef in a large ziplock bag with the arrowroot starch, salt, and pepper until evenly coated. Shake out any excess starch.
- In a big skillet, warm the coconut oil over medium-high heat. Brown the beef on all sides for about 15 minutes. Transfer to a 6-quart slow cooker and set aside.

- In a small mixing bowl, combine the beef bone broth, apple cider vinegar, rosemary, thyme, bay leaves, and garlic. Pour over the beef in the slow cooker and stir to mix.
- Push the carrots, celery, and parsnips down into the liquid.
- Cover and cook on low heat for 8 hours, or until the beef and vegetables are tender.
- Sprinkle with parsley and serve.

## AIP Salmon and Dill Sauce

**Servings: four.**

**Prep time is 10 minutes.**

**Cook for 15 minutes.**

**Ingredients:**

- Four salmon fillets, about six ounces apiece.
- Two tablespoons of olive oil.
- Add salt and pepper to taste.
- A quarter cup of coconut yogurt
- 2 tablespoons fresh dill, chopped
- One tablespoon of lemon juice.
- One-quarter teaspoon of garlic powder

**Instructions:**

- Preheat the oven to 375°F. Use parchment paper to line a baking sheet.
- Arrange the salmon fillets on the prepared baking sheet and drizzle with olive oil. Season with salt and pepper to taste.
- Bake for 15 minutes, or until salmon is flaky and fully cooked.
- In a small bowl, combine the coconut yogurt, dill, lemon juice, and garlic powder. Season with salt and pepper to taste.
- Serve the salmon with the dill sauce and enjoy!

## AIP Pork Chops and Apple Sauce

**Servings: four.**

**Prepare time: 5 minutes.**

**Cook for 20 minutes.**

**Ingredients:**

- 2 tablespoons olive oil.
- Four pork loin chops, center cut (approximately 1 1/4 pounds)
- 1/4 teaspoon sea salt.
- One-fourth of a teaspoon black pepper; remove for AIP

- 2 tablespoons fresh thyme.

- Two tablespoons of fresh rosemary

- Two red apples, cored and sliced

- One-quarter cup chicken broth

- Two tablespoons of apple cider vinegar.

- 2 tablespoons honey.

**Instructions:**

- Heat olive oil in a large skillet over medium-high heat, then season the pork chops with salt and pepper on both sides. Rub the thyme and rosemary all over the pork chops and place them in the skillet.

- Cook for 4 minutes per side, or until golden and heated through. Transfer to a dish to keep heated.

- In the same skillet, combine the apple slices, chicken broth, cider vinegar, and honey.

- Bring to a boil and cook, stirring periodically, until the apples are tender and the sauce has thickened slightly, about 10 minutes.

- Top the pork chops with apple sauce. Enjoy!

# AIP Lamb Kebabs with Cucumber-Herb Relish

**Servings: four.**

**Prep time: 1 hour and 20 minutes.**

**Cook time: 30 minutes**

**Ingredients:**

**For the kebabs:**

- 1 small onion (about 1/4 cup when minced)
- 3–4 sprigs fresh parsley
- One tablespoon of fresh oregano.
- 1/4 teaspoon salt.
- One pound of ground lamb
- Eight metal skewers.

**Regarding the relish:**

- One large cucumber.
- Juice of one lemon
- One tablespoon olive oil.
- 1 tablespoon fresh mint or any herb of your choice.
- Salt to taste.

## Instructions:

- In a food processor, finely chop the onion, parsley, and oregano. Combine salt and ground lamb. Process for up to 1 minute, until a thick paste forms and the onions and herbs are evenly dispersed.

- Remove the meat mixture from the food processor and divide it into eight equal portions. Shape the meat into long cylinders on metal skewers with your hands.

- Refrigerate for at least an hour to let the flavors mingle and the meat firm up.

- Preheat the grill or broiler on high. When the grill is hot, gently set the kebabs on the grate, cover, and cook for 5 minutes without moving.

- Turn the kebabs over and cook for an additional 10 minutes, rotating every 3-4 minutes to ensure browning and grill marks on all sides. Allow the kebabs to rest for 10 minutes and then serve with cucumber relish.

- To create the cucumber relish, peel and dice the cucumber and set it in a small bowl.

- Toss in lemon juice, olive oil, mint, and salt until combined. Refrigerate until ready to serve.

# AIP Shrimp Scampi.

**Servings: four.**

**Prep time is 10 minutes.**

**Cook for 15 minutes.**

**Ingredients:**

- One-quarter cup coconut oil
- 4 garlic cloves, minced
- 1/4 teaspoon red pepper flakes (omit during the elimination phase of AIP)
- One pound of big shrimp, peeled and deveined
- Add salt and pepper to taste.
- Two teaspoons of lemon juice.
- 2 tablespoons chopped parsley.
- Four cups of cooked spaghetti squash.

**Instructions:**

- In a big skillet, warm the coconut oil over medium-high heat. Sauté the garlic and red pepper flakes until fragrant, about 2 minutes.
- Add pepper and salt to taste when preparing the shrimp. Cook for about 10 minutes, stirring periodically, until pink and well cooked.

- Remove from the fire and stir in the parsley and lemon juice.
- Serve the prawns with the spaghetti squash and enjoy!

# AIP Turkey Meatballs

**Servings: four.**

**Prepare time: 15 minutes.**

**Cook for 25 minutes.**

**Ingredients:**

- One pound of ground turkey.
- 1/4 cup chopped fresh parsley.
- Two teaspoons of coconut flour.
- One teaspoon garlic powder.
- One teaspoon of onion powder.
- A half teaspoon of salt.
- 1/4 teaspoon black pepper (omit during the elimination phase of AIP)
- Two teaspoons of coconut oil.
- 2 cups marinara sauce (AIP-compliant)
- Fresh basil to garnish.

**Instructions:**

- In a large mixing bowl, add turkey, parsley, coconut flour, garlic powder, onion powder, salt, and pepper. Mix thoroughly and divide into 16 equal-sized balls.
- Heat the coconut oil in a big skillet over medium-high heat. Brown the meatballs on all sides for about 15 minutes. Transfer to a dish to keep heated.
- In the same skillet, heat the marinara sauce to a boil. Reduce the heat to a simmer for about 10 minutes, or until slightly thickened.
- Return the meatballs to the skillet and coat in the sauce. Simmer for approximately 5 minutes, or until thoroughly heated.
- Sprinkle with basil and serve.

## AIP Chicken Alfredo

**Servings: four.**

**Prepare time: 15 minutes.**

**Cook for 15 minutes.**

**Ingredients:**

- 4 chicken breasts, pounded thin
- Add salt and pepper to taste.

- Two teaspoons of coconut oil.

- One-quarter cup coconut cream

- Two tablespoons of nutritional yeast.

- One-quarter teaspoon of garlic powder

- One-quarter teaspoon of onion powder

- Four cups cooked zucchini noodles.

- Fresh parsley to garnish.

**Instructions:**

- Sprinkle the chicken breasts with salt and pepper on both sides.

- Heat the coconut oil in a big skillet over medium-high heat. Cook the chicken for about 4 minutes on each side, or until brown and cooked through. Transfer to a cutting board and cut thinly. Stay warm.

- In a small saucepan over low heat, combine the coconut cream, nutritional yeast, garlic powder, and onion powder.

- Season with salt and pepper to taste. Cook for approximately 5 minutes, until smooth and bubbling.

- Place the chicken over the zucchini noodles and sprinkle with the sauce. Sprinkle with parsley and enjoy!

# AIP Beef Tacos

**Servings: four.**

**Prepare time: 15 minutes.**

**Cook for 15 minutes.**

**Ingredients:**

*Regarding the tortillas:*

- One-quarter cup coconut flour
- 1/4 cup arrowroot starch.
- One-quarter teaspoon of salt
- One-quarter cup water
- Two teaspoons of coconut oil.

*For the Filling:*

- One tablespoon of coconut oil.
- 1/2 lb. ground beef.
- One-quarter teaspoon of salt
- 1/4 teaspoon black pepper.
- One-quarter teaspoon of garlic powder
- One-quarter teaspoon of onion powder
- 1/4 teaspoon oregano.
- One-quarter teaspoon of cumin
- One-quarter teaspoon of turmeric

- Two cups of shredded lettuce.
- 1/4 cup chopped cilantro.
- A quarter cup of coconut yogurt

**Instructions:**

- To create the tortillas, combine the coconut flour, arrowroot starch, and salt in a medium mixing basin. Add the water and coconut oil, and stir to produce a smooth dough.
- Divide the dough into eight equal sections, then roll each into a ball. Place each ball between two sheets of parchment paper and use a rolling pin or your hands to flatten into a thin circle.
- In a non-stick skillet over medium heat, cook each tortilla for about 2 minutes on each side, or until lightly browned and cooked through. Transfer to a dish to keep heated.
- To make the filling, in a big skillet, warm the coconut oil over medium-high heat. Cook the beef, breaking it up with a spatula, until browned and cooked through, about 15 minutes.
- Drain out any extra fat and season with salt, pepper, garlic powder, onion powder, oregano, cumin, and turmeric. Stir thoroughly to mix.

- To make the tacos, put part of the beef mixture onto each tortilla, then top with lettuce, cilantro, and coconut yogurt. Fold in half and enjoy!

# AIP Lemon Garlic Shrimp

**Servings: four.**

**Prep time is 10 minutes.**

**Cook for 10 minutes.**

**Ingredients:**

- One-quarter cup coconut oil
- 4 garlic cloves, minced
- One-quarter teaspoon of salt
- 1/4 teaspoon black pepper (omit during the elimination phase of AIP)
- One pound of big shrimp, peeled and deveined
- Two teaspoons of lemon juice.
- 2 tablespoons chopped parsley.
- Four cups cooked cauliflower rice.

**Instructions**:

- In a big skillet, warm the coconut oil over medium-high heat. Sauté the garlic, salt, and pepper until fragrant, about 2 minutes.
- Cook the shrimp, tossing regularly, until pink and cooked through, about 10 minutes.
- Remove from the fire and stir in the parsley and lemon juice.
- Serve the shrimp with cauliflower rice and enjoy!

# CHAPTER 7

## Side Dishes

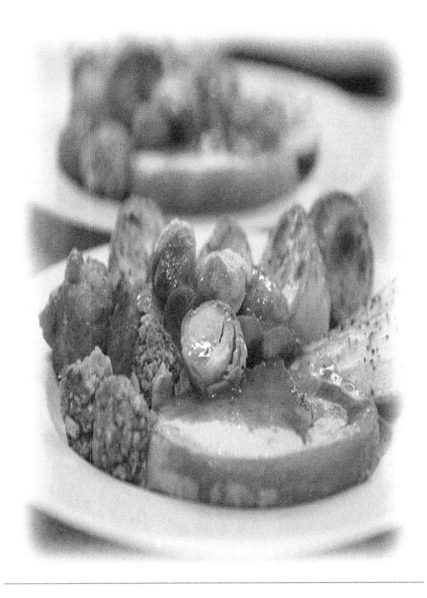

# AIP Roasted Brussels sprouts

**Servings: four.**

**Prep time is 10 minutes.**

**Cook for 25 minutes.**

**Ingredients:**

- 1 pound of trimmed and halved Brussels sprouts.
- Two teaspoons of heated coconut oil.
- Add salt and pepper to taste.

**Instructions:**

- Preheat the oven to 400°F. Use parchment paper to line a baking sheet.
- Toss the Brussels sprouts with the coconut oil, salt, and pepper, then arrange them evenly on the prepared baking sheet.
- Roast for 25 minutes, until crisp and brown, stirring halfway through.
- Enjoy your easy yet wonderful side dish!

# AIP Mashed Cauliflower

**Servings: four.**

**Prep time is 10 minutes.**

**Cook for 15 minutes.**

**Ingredients:**

- Cut 1 large head of cauliflower into florets.
- Four cups of water.
- One-quarter cup coconut cream
- 2 tablespoons of ghee (or coconut oil for the vegan version).
- Add salt and pepper to taste.
- Fresh parsley to garnish.

**Instructions:**

- Bring a large saucepan of water to a boil, then add the cauliflower florets. Cook for approximately 15 minutes, or until tender. Drain thoroughly and transfer to a big bowl.
- Use a potato masher or immersion blender to mash the cauliflower until smooth and creamy.
- Stir in the coconut cream, ghee, salt, and pepper, and season to taste.
- Sprinkle with parsley and serve.

# AIP Sweet Potato Fries

**Servings: four.**

**Prep time is 10 minutes.**

**Cook for 25 minutes.**

**Ingredients**:

- Two large sweet potatoes, peeled and sliced into thin wedges
- Two teaspoons of heated coconut oil.
- Add salt and pepper to taste.

**Instructions:**

- Preheat the oven to 425°F. Use parchment paper to line a baking sheet.
- Toss the sweet potato wedges with the coconut oil, salt, and pepper, then arrange in a single layer on the prepared baking sheet.
- Bake until golden and crisp, about 25 minutes. Flip halfway through.
- Enjoy your crispy, sweet side dish!

# AIP Zucchini Noodles

**Servings: four.**

**Prep time is 10 minutes.**

**Cook for 10 minutes.**

**• Ingredients:**

- 4 medium zucchinis spiralized or peeled into thin ribbons.
- Two teaspoons of coconut oil.
- Add salt and pepper to taste.
- Fresh basil to garnish.

**Instructions**:

- In a big skillet, warm the coconut oil over medium-high heat. Sauté the zucchini noodles for about 10 minutes, or until soft. Season with salt and pepper to taste.
- Sprinkle with basil and serve.

# AIP Roasted Beets

**Servings: four.**

**Prep time is 10 minutes.**

**Cook for 45 minutes.**

**Ingredients:**

- Four medium beets, peeled and chopped
- Two teaspoons of heated coconut oil.
- Add salt and pepper to taste.

**Instructions:**

- \
- Preheat the oven to 375°F. Use parchment paper to line a baking sheet.
- Toss the beets with the coconut oil, salt, and pepper, then distribute them evenly on the prepared baking sheet.
- Roast until tender and caramelized, about 45 minutes. Stir halfway through.
- Enjoy this colorful and healthful side dish!

# AIP Baked Plantains

**Servings: four.**

**Prepare time: 5 minutes.**

**Cook for 25 minutes.**

**Ingredients:**

- Four ripe plantains, peeled and sliced
- Two teaspoons of heated coconut oil.
- Two teaspoons of honey.
- One-fourth teaspoon cinnamon

**Instructions:**

- Preheat the oven to 375°F. Use parchment paper to line a baking sheet.
- In a small bowl, combine the coconut oil, honey, and cinnamon.
- Place the plantain slices on the prepared baking sheet and brush them with the honey mixture.
- Bake for 25 minutes, or until golden and tender. Flip halfway through.
- Enjoy your sweet, tropical side dish!

# AIP Garlic Green Beans

**Servings: four.**

**Prep time is 10 minutes.**

**Cook for 15 minutes.**

**Ingredients:**

- One pound of trimmed green beans
- Two teaspoons of coconut oil.
- 4 garlic cloves, minced
- Add salt and pepper to taste.

**Instructions:**

- Blanch the green beans in a large pot of boiling water for 5 minutes, or until they are crisp tender. To halt the cooking process, drain and rinse well with cold water.
- In a big skillet, warm the coconut oil over medium-high heat. Sauté the garlic until fragrant, about 2 minutes.
- Stir in the green beans and season with salt and pepper to taste. Cook for approximately 10 minutes, stirring periodically, until thoroughly cooked.
- Enjoy your garlicky, crispy side dish!

# AIP Roasted Carrots

**Servings: four.**

**Prep time is 10 minutes.**

**Cook for 25 minutes.**

**Ingredients:**

- 1 pound of carrots, peeled and chopped into 1-inch pieces
- Two teaspoons of heated coconut oil.
- Add salt and pepper to taste.
- 2 tablespoons chopped parsley.

**Instructions:**

- Preheat the oven to 400°F. Use parchment paper to line a baking sheet.
- Toss the carrots with the coconut oil, salt, and pepper, then arrange them evenly on the prepared baking sheet.
- Roast for 25 minutes, or until soft and caramelized. Stir halfway through.
- Sprinkle with parsley and serve.

# AIP Cauliflower Rice

**Servings: four.**

**Prep time is 10 minutes.**

**Cook for 10 minutes.**

**Ingredients:**

- Cut 1 large head of cauliflower into florets.
- Two teaspoons of coconut oil.
- Add salt and pepper to taste.

**Instructions**:

- Using a food processor, pulse the cauliflower florets until they resemble rice. You might need to perform this in batches.
- Heat the coconut oil in a big skillet over medium-high heat.
- Sauté the cauliflower rice for about 10 minutes, or until cooked. Season with salt and pepper to taste.
- Savor your low-carb, grain-free side dish!

# AIP Sautéed Spinach

**Servings: four.**

**Prep time is 10 minutes.**

**Cook for 10 minutes.**

**Ingredients:**

- Two teaspoons of coconut oil.
- 4 garlic cloves, minced
- Eight cups of fresh spinach.
- Add salt and pepper to taste.
- Two teaspoons of lemon juice.

**Instructions:**

- In a big skillet, warm the coconut oil over medium-high heat. Sauté the garlic until fragrant, about 2 minutes.
- Stir in the spinach and season with salt and pepper to taste. Cook for approximately 10 minutes, stirring periodically, until wilted.
- Drizzle with lemon juice and serve.

# CHAPTER 8

## Snack and Treat

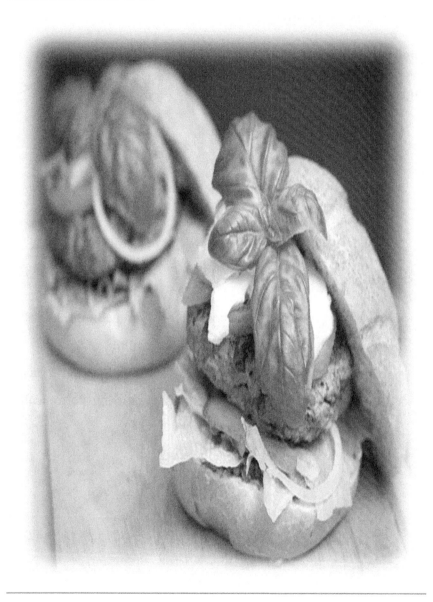

# AIP Banana Bread

**Serves: 8**

**Prep time is 10 minutes.**

**Cook for 50 minutes.**

**Ingredients:**

- 4 ripe bananas (mashed)
- 1/4 cup melted coconut oil.
- One-quarter cup honey
- One teaspoon of vanilla extract.
- One-quarter cup coconut flour
- 1/4 cup arrowroot starch.
- One-half teaspoon of baking soda
- One-quarter teaspoon of salt
- One-fourth teaspoon cinnamon

**Instructions:**

- Preheat the oven to 350°F. Line a 9x5-inch loaf pan with parchment paper.
- In a large mixing bowl, blend the bananas, coconut oil, honey, and vanilla essence until thoroughly incorporated.
- In a small bowl, combine the coconut flour, arrowroot starch, baking soda, salt, and cinnamon.

- Combine the dry ingredients with the wet components and mix thoroughly to produce a homogeneous batter.
- After adding the mixture to the loaf pan that has been ready, level the top with a spatula.
- A toothpick put into the center should come out clean after baking for 50 minutes.
- Allow the bread to completely cool in the pan before slicing and serving.

## AIP Coconut Cookies

**Serves: 12**

**Prepare time: 15 minutes.**

**Cook for 15 minutes.**

**Ingredients:**

- 1/4 cup of softened coconut oil
- One-quarter cup honey
- One teaspoon of vanilla extract.
- One-quarter teaspoon of salt
- 1 1/2 cups unsweetened shredded coconut.
- Two teaspoons of coconut flour.

**Instructions**:

- Preheat the oven to 350°F. Use parchment paper to line a baking sheet.
- Use an electric mixer to cream the coconut oil, honey, vanilla extract, and salt in a large bowl until frothy.
- Combine the shredded coconut and coconut flour, mixing thoroughly to produce a sticky dough.
- Drop by rounded tablespoonfuls onto the prepared baking sheet, leaving some space between each.
- Gently flatten the cookies with your fingertips or a spatula.
- Bake for 15 minutes, or until golden and firm around the edges.
- Cool the cookies on the baking sheet for 10 minutes before transferring to a wire rack to cool fully.

# AIP Apple Chips

**Servings: four.**

**Prep time is 10 minutes.**

**Cooking time: 2 hours.**

**Ingredients:**

- Two large apples, cored and thinly sliced
- One-fourth teaspoon cinnamon

**Instructions**:

- Preheat the oven to 200°F. Line two baking pans with parchment paper.
- Place the apple slices in a single layer on the prepared baking pans, then sprinkle with cinnamon.
- Bake for 2 hours, or until crisp and dry. Flip halfway through.
- Allow the apple chips to completely cool on the baking sheets before storing in an airtight container.

# AIP Carrot Cake

**Serves: 9**

**Prepare time: 15 minutes.**

**Cook for 25 minutes.**

**Ingredients:**

*For the Cake:*

- 1/4 cup melted coconut oil.
- One-quarter cup honey
- 1/4 cup unsweetened applesauce.
- One teaspoon of vanilla extract.
- One-quarter cup coconut flour
- 1/4 cup arrowroot starch.
- One-half teaspoon of baking soda
- One-quarter teaspoon of salt
- One-fourth teaspoon cinnamon
- One-quarter teaspoon ginger
- 1/4 teaspoon nutmeg.
- 1 cup shredded carrots.

## For frosting:

- 1/4 cup softened coconut butter.
- Two teaspoons of honey.
- Two teaspoons of coconut cream.
- One-quarter teaspoon of vanilla extract
- One-quarter teaspoon of lemon juice

## Instructions:

- To make the cake, preheat the oven to 350°F and butter an 8x8 baking pan.
- In a large mixing basin, blend the coconut oil, honey, applesauce, and vanilla essence until thoroughly incorporated.
- In a small bowl, combine the coconut flour, arrowroot starch, baking soda, salt, cinnamon, ginger, and nutmeg.
- Combine the dry ingredients with the wet components and mix thoroughly to produce a homogeneous batter.
- Fold in the grated carrots and equally distribute the batter in the prepared baking pan.
- A toothpick put into the center should come out clean after 25 minutes of baking.
- Allow the cake to completely cool in the pan before icing.

- In a small bowl, combine the coconut butter, honey, coconut cream, vanilla essence, and lemon juice. Whisk until smooth and creamy.
- Spread the icing on the cooled cake and cut into nine squares. Enjoy!

# AIP Pumpkin Muffins

**Serves: 12**

**Prep time is 10 minutes.**

**Cook for 25 minutes.**

**Ingredients:**

- 1/4 cup melted coconut oil.
- One-quarter cup honey
- 4 eggs
- 1 cup pumpkin puree.
- One teaspoon of vanilla extract.
- One-quarter cup coconut flour
- 1/4 cup arrowroot starch.
- One-half teaspoon of baking soda
- One-quarter teaspoon of salt
- One teaspoon of cinnamon.

- 1/4 teaspoon nutmeg.

**Instructions**:

- Preheat the oven to 350°F. Line a 12-cup muffin tray with paper liners.
- In a large mixing bowl, blend the coconut oil, honey, eggs, pumpkin puree, and vanilla essence until thoroughly incorporated.
- In a small bowl, combine the coconut flour, arrowroot starch, baking soda, salt, cinnamon, and nutmeg.
- Combine the dry ingredients with the wet components and mix thoroughly to produce a homogeneous batter.
- Divide the batter evenly among the prepared muffin cups, filling each about 3/4 full.
- A toothpick put into the center should come out clean after 25 minutes of baking.
- Allow the muffins to cool briefly in the pan before transferring to a wire rack to cool entirely.

# AIP Berry Parfait.

**Servings: four.**

**Prep time is 10 minutes.**

**Ingredients:**

- Two cups of coconut yogurt.
- Two cups of mixed berries, including strawberries, blueberries, raspberries, and blackberries.
- 1/4 cup unsweetened shredded coconut.
- Two teaspoons of honey.

**Instructions**:

- In a small bowl, combine the berries and honey and leave aside.
- In four glasses or jars, layer the coconut yogurt, berry mixture, and shredded coconut, repeating until all of the ingredients are utilized.
- Enjoy your creamy, fruity treat!

# AIP Cinnamon Apple Crisp

**Servings: six.**

**Prepare time: 15 minutes.**

**Cook for 35 minutes.**

**Ingredients:**

*For the Filling:*

- 4 big apples, peeled, cored, and sliced
- Two teaspoons of lemon juice.
- Two teaspoons of honey.
- One teaspoon of cinnamon.

*For the toppings:*

- 1/4 cup melted coconut oil.
- One-quarter cup honey
- One-quarter cup coconut flour
- 1/4 cup arrowroot starch.
- One-quarter teaspoon of salt
- One-fourth teaspoon cinnamon
- 1/4 cup unsweetened shredded coconut.

**Instructions**:

- To prepare the filling, preheat the oven to 375°F and butter an 8x8 baking dish.
- In a large bowl, combine the apple slices, lemon juice, honey, and cinnamon. Transfer to the prepared baking dish and distribute evenly.
- In a small bowl, combine the coconut oil, honey, coconut flour, arrowroot starch, salt, and cinnamon. Add the shredded coconut and crumble the mixture over the apple layer.
- Bake for 35 minutes, or until the apples bubble and the topping is golden and crunchy.
- Before serving, let the crisp to cool slightly.

# AIP Lemon Bars

**Serves: 9**

**Prepare time: 15 minutes.**

**Cook for 25 minutes.**

**Ingredients:**

*For the crust:*

- 1/4 cup melted coconut oil.
- One-quarter cup honey
- One-quarter teaspoon of salt
- One-quarter cup coconut flour
- 1/4 cup arrowroot starch.

*For the Filling:*

- 4 eggs
- 1/2 cup honey.
- 1/2 cup lemon juice.
- Two teaspoons of coconut flour.
- 1/4 teaspoon of turmeric (for coloring)
- Dust with powdered coconut sugar (optional).

**Instructions:**

- Preheat the oven to 350°F and prepare an 8x8-inch baking tray with parchment paper.
- In a large basin, combine the coconut oil, honey, and salt. Mix in the coconut flour and arrowroot starch until the dough comes together.
- Press the dough evenly onto the prepared baking sheet and bake for 10 minutes, or until gently brown.
- In a medium bowl, combine the eggs, honey, lemon juice, coconut flour, and turmeric. Whisk until smooth and frothy.
- Spread the filling over the hot crust and bake for 15 minutes, or until set in the center.
- Allow the bars to cool completely in the pan before cutting into nine squares. Sprinkle with powdered coconut sugar if preferred, and enjoy!

# AIP Chocolate Chip Cookies

**Serves: 12**

**Prepare time: 15 minutes.**

**Cook for 15 minutes.**

**Ingredients:**

- 1/4 cup of softened coconut oil
- One-quarter cup honey
- One teaspoon of vanilla extract.
- One-quarter teaspoon of salt
- One-quarter cup coconut flour
- 1/4 cup carob powder.
- 1/4 cup handmade chocolate chips (see to remark below).

**Instructions:**

- Preheat the oven to 350°F. Use parchment paper to line a baking sheet.
- Use an electric mixer to cream the coconut oil, honey, vanilla extract, and salt in a large bowl until frothy.
- Combine the coconut flour and carob powder, mixing thoroughly to produce a sticky dough.

- Fold in the chocolate chips and place rounded tablespoonful on the prepared baking sheet, allowing some space between them.
- Gently flatten the cookies with your fingertips or a spatula.
- Bake for 15 minutes, until the edges are crisp.
- Cool the cookies on the baking sheet for 10 minutes before transferring to a wire rack to cool fully.
- To make homemade chocolate chips, combine 1/4 cup coconut oil and 1/4 cup carob powder in a small saucepan over low heat.
- Stir until smooth. Mix in 2 tablespoons honey and a teaspoon of salt. Pour the mixture into a small baking dish lined with parchment paper and freeze for approximately 15 minutes.
- Cut into small pieces and freeze until ready for use.

# CHAPTER 9

## Sauces & Dressings

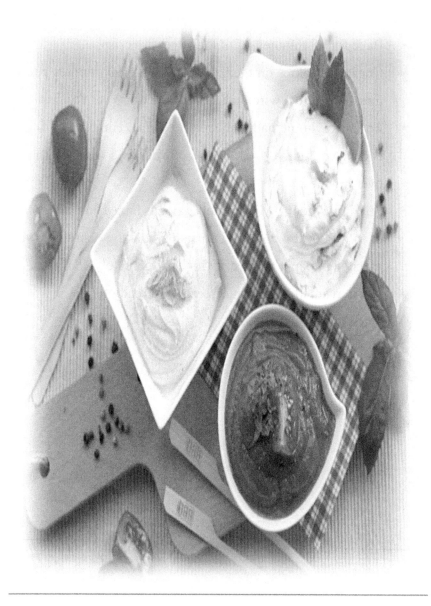

# AIP Barbeque Sauce

**Servings: approximately 2 cups.**

**Prep time is 10 minutes.**

**Ingredients:**

- 1 cup + 2 tablespoons nomato sauce (recipe below)
- 1/4 cup coconut aminos.
- Three tablespoons blackstrap molasses.
- One tablespoon balsamic vinegar.
- 2 tbsp and 1 tsp apple cider vinegar
- One teaspoon of onion powder
- 1/2 teaspoon garlic powder.
- 1/2 teaspoon sea salt.
- 1/4 cup of minced parsley.
- 1/2 tbsp chopped fresh dill.
- 1/4 tsp black pepper (omit during the AIP elimination phase).

**Instructions:**

- Place all of the ingredients in a high-speed blender and blend until well combined. Taste the sauce and season as desired, or add water to make it thinner.
- Store in the fridge in a glass container for 3-4 days (or freeze) and use as a BBQ sauce substitute.

# Nomato Sauce

**Servings: approximately 2 cups.**

**Prepare time: 30 minutes.**

**Ingredients:**

- One tablespoon olive oil.
- One-quarter cup chopped onion
- 2 garlic cloves, minced
- 2 cups of peeled and chopped butternut squash.
- One tiny beet, peeled and diced
- 2 cups chicken bone broth (or vegetable broth if vegan)
- Two tablespoons dried basil.
- One tablespoon of dried oregano.
- One teaspoon of dried rosemary
- 1/4 teaspoon sea salt.
- 2 tablespoons red wine vinegar.

**Instructions:**

- Heat the oil in a big pot on medium-high heat. Cook the onion and garlic, stirring regularly, until softened, about 10 minutes.
- Heat the squash, beet, broth, basil, oregano, rosemary, and salt until boiling. Cook, covered, until the squash and beets are soft, about 20 minutes.

- In a blender, combine the ingredients and process until smooth. After adding the vinegar, taste and adjust the seasoning.
- Refrigerate in glass for up to a week, or freeze for later use.

## AIP Ranch Dressing

**Servings: approximately 1 cup.**

**Prepare time: 5 minutes.**

**Ingredients:**

- 1/2 cup of full-fat coconut milk
- 1/4 cup plain coconut yogurt.
- 2 tablespoons avocado oil.
- One tablespoon of apple cider vinegar.
- One teaspoon of onion powder
- 1/2 teaspoon garlic powder.
- 1/2 teaspoon sea salt.
- 2 tablespoons chopped fresh parsley
- 1 tsp freshly chopped dill.

**Instructions**:

- In a small bowl, whisk together the coconut milk, coconut yogurt, avocado oil, and apple cider vinegar.
- Add the onion powder, garlic powder, salt, parsley, and dill.
- Refrigerate in glass containers for up to a week and serve as a salad dressing or dip.

## AIP Avocado Mayo

**Servings: approximately 1 cup.**

**Prep time is 10 minutes.**

**Ingredients:**

- One ripe avocado, peeled and pitted
- One-quarter cup olive oil
- 2 tablespoons lemon juice.
- 1/4 teaspoon sea salt.
- 1/4 teaspoon garlic powder.

**Instructions**:

- In a blender or food processor, combine the avocado, olive oil, lemon juice, salt, and garlic powder. Puree until smooth and creamy, scraping down the sides as needed.

- Refrigerate in a glass container for up to three days and use as a mayonnaise alternative.

# AIP Honey Mustard Dressing

**Servings: approximately 1/2 cup.**

**Prepare time: 5 minutes.**

**Ingredients:**

- One-quarter cup coconut cream
- 2 tablespoons honey.
- Two tablespoons of apple cider vinegar.
- One teaspoon of onion powder
- 1/2 teaspoon ginger powder.
- 1/4 teaspoon sea salt.

**Instructions:**

- In a small bowl, whisk together all of the ingredients until thoroughly blended.
- Refrigerate in glass containers for up to a week and serve as a salad dressing or dip.

# AIP Tomato Sauce

**Servings: approximately 2 cups.**

**Prepare time: 30 minutes.**

**Ingredients:**

- One tablespoon olive oil.
- One-quarter cup chopped onion
- 2 garlic cloves, minced
- 2 cups of peeled and chopped butternut squash.
- One tiny beet, peeled and diced
- 2 cups chicken bone broth (or vegetable broth if vegan)
- Two tablespoons dried basil.
- One tablespoon of dried oregano.
- One teaspoon of dried rosemary
- 1/4 teaspoon sea salt.
- 2 tablespoons red wine vinegar.

**Instructions:**

- Proceed in the same manner as the nomato sauce recipe above.

# AIP Pesto Sauce

**Servings: approximately 1 cup.**

**Prepare time: 15 minutes.**

**Ingredients:**

- 1.5 cups chopped fresh basil, loosely packed
- 1/2 cup of chopped fresh spinach, lightly packed.
- 5 garlic cloves, peeled and chopped
- One-quarter cup olive oil
- 2 tablespoons lemon juice.
- 1/4 teaspoon sea salt.

**Instructions:**

- Combine all of the ingredients in a blender or food processor; blend until smooth and creamy, scraping down the sides as needed.
- Refrigerate for up to a week in a glass container and serve as a sauce with pasta, chicken, fish, or vegetables.

# AIP Caesar Dressing

**Servings: approximately 1 cup.**

**Prep time is 10 minutes.**

**Ingredients:**

- One-quarter cup coconut cream
- 2 tablespoons nutritional yeast.
- 2 tablespoons lemon juice.
- 2 teaspoons anchovy paste
- 1 teaspoon Dijon mustard
- One teaspoon garlic powder.
- 1/4 teaspoon sea salt.
- 1/4 tsp black pepper (omit during the AIP elimination phase).
- One-quarter cup olive oil

**Instructions:**

- In a blender or food processor, combine all of the ingredients except the olive oil. Blend until smooth and creamy, scraping down the sides as needed.
- While the blender or food processor is running, slowly trickle in the olive oil until fully combined.
- Refrigerate in glass containers for up to a week and serve as a salad dressing or dip.

# AIP Teriyaki Sauce

**Servings: approximately 1/2 cup.**

**Prep time is 10 minutes.**

**Ingredients:**

- 1/4 cup coconut aminos.
- 2 tablespoons honey.
- Two tablespoons of apple cider vinegar.
- One teaspoon of ginger powder.
- 1/2 teaspoon garlic powder.
- 1/4 teaspoon sea salt.
- One tablespoon of arrowroot starch.
- 2 tablespoons water.

**Instructions:**

- In a small saucepan over medium-high heat, combine the coconut aminos, honey, vinegar, ginger, garlic, and salt.
- Bring to a boil, then turn down the heat and simmer for 5 minutes, stirring regularly.
- In a small mixing bowl, combine the arrowroot starch and water. Whisk until smooth. Add the slurry to the pot and stir until combined.
- Cook for a further 5 minutes, stirring often, until the sauce is thick and glossy.

- Refrigerate in glass containers for up to a week and use as a sauce for chicken, beef, pork, or vegetables.

## AIP Salsa Verde

**Servings: approximately 2 cups.**

**Prep time is 20 minutes.**

**Ingredients:**

- 1 lb of tomatillos, husked and washed
- One-quarter cup chopped onion
- 2 garlic cloves, peeled
- 1/4 cup of chopped cilantro.
- 2 tablespoons lime juice.
- 1/2 teaspoon sea salt.
- 1/4 tsp cumin (omit for elimination phase of AIP).

**Instructions:**

- Cut the tomatillos in quarters and arrange in a large pot. Cover with water and bring to a boil.
- Reduce the heat and let the tomatillos simmer for about 15 minutes, or until softened. Drain and allow to cool somewhat.

- Place the tomatillos in a blender or food processor. Add the onion, garlic, cilantro, lime juice, salt, and cumin (if using).
- Blend until smooth and creamy, scraping down the sides as necessary.
- Refrigerate in glass for up to a week and use as a dip, sauce, or marinade.

# AIP Chimichurri Sauce

**Servings: approximately 1 cup.**

**Prepare time: 5 minutes.**

**Ingredients:**

- 1 cup of cilantro, packed tightly
- 1/4 cup of parsley, neatly packed
- 2 garlic cloves, peeled and chopped
- One-quarter cup olive oil
- Two tablespoons of apple cider vinegar.
- 1/2 teaspoon sea salt.
- 1/4 tsp red pepper flakes (omit for elimination phase of AIP)

**Instructions**:

- Add all of the ingredients to a blender or food processor and pulse until finely chopped, scraping down the sides as needed.
- Refrigerate in a glass container for up to a week and use as a sauce for grilled meats, seafood, or vegetables.

## 2-Week Meal Plan

**Week 1:**

*Day 1:*

- Breakfast: AIP Green Smoothie
- Lunch: AIP Chicken Soup with AIP Roasted Brussels Sprouts
- Dinner: AIP Chicken Stir Fry with AIP Mashed Cauliflower
- Snack: AIP Banana Bread

*Day 2:*

- Breakfast: Coconut Flour Pancakes
- Lunch: AIP Broccoli Soup with AIP Sweet Potato Fries
- Dinner: AIP Beef Stew with AIP Zucchini Noodles
- Snack: AIP Coconut Cookies

*Day 3:*

- Breakfast: Sweet Potato Hash
- Lunch: AIP Pumpkin Soup with AIP Roasted Beets
- Dinner: AIP Salmon with Dill Sauce with AIP Baked Plantains
- Snack: AIP Apple Chips

*Day 4:*

- Breakfast: AIP Breakfast Casserole
- Lunch: AIP Salad with Grilled Chicken with AIP Garlic Green Beans
- Dinner: AIP Pork Chops with Apple Sauce with AIP Roasted Carrots
- Snack: AIP Carrot Cake

*Day 5:*

- Breakfast: Banana Cinnamon Muffins
- Lunch: AIP Greek Salad with AIP Cauliflower Rice
- Dinner: AIP Lamb Kebabs with AIP Sautéed Spinach
- Snack: AIP Zucchini Bread

*Day 6:*

- Breakfast: AIP Porridge
- Lunch: AIP Coleslaw with AIP Roasted Brussels Sprouts
- Dinner: AIP Shrimp Scampi with AIP Mashed Cauliflower
- Snack: AIP Pumpkin Muffins

*Day 7:*

- Breakfast: Sausage and Veggie Skillet
- Lunch: AIP Kale Salad with AIP Sweet Potato Fries
- Dinner: AIP Turkey Meatballs with AIP Zucchini Noodles
- Snack: AIP Berry Parfait

**Week 2:**

*Day 8:*

- Breakfast: AIP Breakfast Tacos
- Lunch: AIP Beetroot Soup with AIP Roasted Beets
- Dinner: AIP Chicken Alfredo with AIP Baked Plantains
- Snack: AIP Cinnamon Apple Crisp

*Day 9:*

- Breakfast: AIP Waffles
- Lunch: AIP Cucumber Salad with AIP Garlic Green Beans
- Dinner: AIP Beef Tacos with AIP Roasted Carrots

- Snack: AIP Lemon Bars

*Day 10:*

- Breakfast: AIP Breakfast Burrito
- Lunch: AIP Carrot Soup with AIP Cauliflower Rice
- Dinner: AIP Lemon Garlic Shrimp with AIP Sautéed Spinach
- Snack: AIP Chocolate Chip Cookies

*Day 11:*

- Breakfast: AIP Green Smoothie
- Lunch: AIP Chicken Soup with AIP Roasted Brussels Sprouts
- Dinner: AIP Chicken Stir Fry with AIP Mashed Cauliflower
- Snack: AIP Banana Bread

*Day 12:*

- Breakfast: Coconut Flour Pancakes
- Lunch: AIP Broccoli Soup with AIP Sweet Potato Fries
- Dinner: AIP Beef Stew with AIP Zucchini Noodles
- Snack: AIP Coconut Cookies

*Day 13:*

- Breakfast: Sweet Potato Hash
- Lunch: AIP Pumpkin Soup with AIP Roasted Beets
- Dinner: AIP Salmon with Dill Sauce with AIP Baked Plantains
- Snack: AIP Apple Chips

*Day 14:*

- Breakfast: AIP Breakfast Casserole
- Lunch: AIP Salad with Grilled Chicken with AIP Garlic Green Beans
- Dinner: AIP Pork Chops with Apple Sauce with AIP Roasted Carrots
- Snack: AIP Carrot Cake

**Remember to use the sauces and dressings from Chapter 9 to add flavour to your meals. Enjoy your meals!**

# CONCLUSION

As you finish the chapters of the Hashimoto AIP Cookbook, I want to express my heartfelt appreciation for joining me on this path to improved health. Remember, this is more than simply a cookbook; it's a guide to a way of life that values both health and flavor.

Encourage yourself and others around you to constantly follow the Hashimoto's AIP lifestyle. Small, consistent steps lay the way for long-term improvement. Your health is worth every tasty option.

While these pages provide helpful insights, it is critical to acknowledge the uniqueness of your health path. Consult a healthcare expert for individualized counsel geared to your specific needs. Your health is your most valuable possession; give it the attention it deserves.

Finally, if the Hashimoto AIP Cookbook has favorably impacted your life, please consider sharing your opinions. Your opinion is more than simply a review; it serves as a beacon for others pursuing a healthier lifestyle. Drop me a line, share your experience, and let's continue to encourage and support one another on this path to bright health.

With Great Gratitude,

Christiana White

Made in United States
Orlando, FL
29 September 2024

52084039R00065